GW00503576

strip

tease

the naughty girl's guide

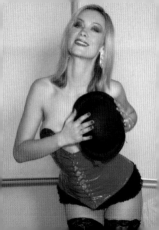

strip
tease

the naughty girl's guide

REBECCA DRURY

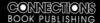
CONNECTIONS
BOOK PUBLISHING

A CONNECTIONS EDITION
This edition published in Great Britain in 2007 by
Connections Book Publishing Limited
St Chad's House, 148 King's Cross Road
London WC1X 9DH
www.connections-publishing.com

British Library Cataloguing-in-Publication data available on request.

ISBN 978-1-85906-209-8

1   3   5   7   9 10 8   6   4   2

Phototypeset in Myriad using QuarkXPress on Apple Macintosh
Printed in Singapore

contents

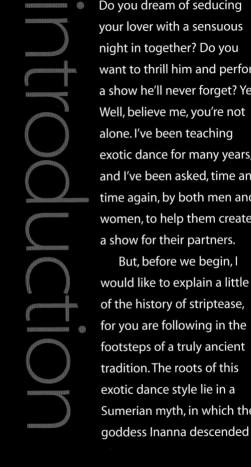

Do you dream of seducing your lover with a sensuous night in together? Do you want to thrill him and perform a show he'll never forget? Yes? Well, believe me, you're not alone. I've been teaching exotic dance for many years, and I've been asked, time and time again, by both men and women, to help them create a show for their partners.

But, before we begin, I would like to explain a little of the history of striptease, for you are following in the footsteps of a truly ancient tradition. The roots of this exotic dance style lie in a Sumerian myth, in which the goddess Inanna descended

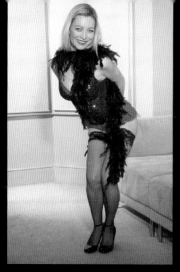

In the New Testament, Salome performed this dance for King Herod. In 1896, Oscar Wilde produced a play called *Salome*, which was then transformed into an opera by Richard Strauss in 1905. These works were what really began the craze that we recognize today as striptease. This in turn has directly influenced exotic dance styles such as lap dancing, Neo Burlesque and pole dancing.

into hell to rescue her lover Damouz. At each of the seven gates she removed a veil and a jewel. As long as she stayed in hell, the earth remained barren, but, when she returned home, fertility prevailed. Inanna's ordeal became known as The Dance of the Seven Veils.

The evolution of striptease has mirrored western society's attitudes towards the female body throughout the last two centuries. Thankfully, today, we can all enjoy a taste of erotic freedom, especially in the

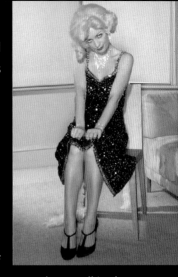

privacy of our own homes, and in this book you'll find all kinds of handy tips and instructions to help you create a fabulous show for you both to enjoy.

For your special night in to be truly spectacular, you'll need to do some preparation. This is the most important part of the show – if you get it right the rest will follow; but, if you don't your performance could fall flat, even if you do know all the dance moves. So, before you start taking off your clothes, take a moment to read part one, Preparation. Here, you'll learn all you need to know about making a date, choosing outfits, creating a passionate environment for your show – all in the name of embracing the age-old tradition of striptease.

There is much more to striptease than simply taking your clothes off; there is an attitude and a style that you should practise before you perform. In the next section, called In the Mood, you will discover how to use your face to entice your lover, how to remove your clothes elegantly and sensuously, how to make effective use of props in your show, and much, much more.

Of course, striptease is a form of dance, so you'll need to learn some moves. First I shall teach you some basic steps that will allow you to make great use of your music as you strip. Each dance move is easy to learn, so you'll be able to concentrate on thrilling your man! To help you add a unique touch to your routine, I shall also show you how to incorporate a chair into your performance. Please give these techniques a go. When performed with style, they are truly wonderful.

To show you how you can bring together all that you've learned, I've choreographed a great little routine for you to try. It's designed purely to give you some ideas, and, when you've mastered it, I hope you'll feel inspired to make up some different ones, and even add some new steps. Make the dance your own – it's going to be performed in *your* home, for *your* lover, after all.

I can't wait for you to get started. If you read this little book from cover to cover, you'll be well on your way to having some of the best nights in of your life.

preparation

You don't have to be the best dancer in the world to put on a great exotic-dance show – but it does help to be prepared. In this section I will guide you through every aspect of planning for your special night.

You'll be amazed at how easy it is to create a sensual atmosphere. With just a sprinkling of imagination and a dash of advice from me, you'll soon have your lover panting with desire!

Discover together the joys of making a date. Watch the longing in your partner's eyes intensify as the big day gets ever closer. For you, the anticipation will be even stronger, as you'll be choosing your clothes and props and practising your dance moves. Ask him to help you create a lovely sensual space in which to perform. You will both enjoy your night in so much more if the environment is just right.

For an extra-special touch, you may like to give yourself a new persona, with a fantasy name – tease your man with your mystique. What will the new you wear? Shhh, don't tell him.

The pulses are racing already, and we haven't even started to dance yet!

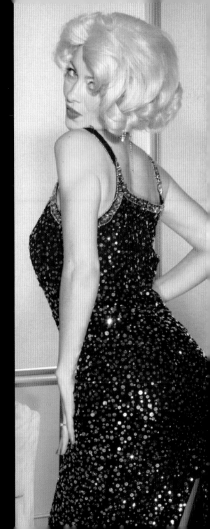

Remember the days when dates were pure agony? The hours before a rendezvous seemed to last for an eternity. These are the feelings we want to rekindle. So, begin by making a date with your lover. Think of the excitement ahead – shopping for your outfit, having your hair done, dreaming about him …

Allow plenty of time to prepare – ideally, about two weeks. Talk about the night together. Ask your man if he has any wishes for the evening. This is a great chance to find out all his hidden fantasies. Who knows *what* he'll suggest!

During the build-up, try to rehearse as much as you can. Whenever your partner is out of the way, practise in the area of the home you intend to use on the night. Try out your costume. Is it easy to take off? Could anything go wrong? If you foresee any problems, now is the time to work out ways to avoid them.

If you feel nervous about your show, express this to your lover. Hopefully, he will put you at your ease by telling you how much he's looking forward to it. It's quite likely that he's feeling a little nervous, too.

It's been said that a great striptease is a game of smoke and mirrors – by creating a flattering environment, you can add a little illusion to your show.

Begin by giving the room a real spring clean. Clear away anything that will remind you of your daily routines. Get your partner to help you tidy up and prepare the scene – you shouldn't have to do everything!

Make your dance area as large as possible, and ensure that any props you intend to use are set up in the right position.

Lighting

It is essential that your dance space is lit in a flattering way, so choose your lighting very carefully. Red lights are sexy, but they can be too dark if used exclusively. However, if they are combined with some soft white lights they could give the ideal effect. Twinkling fairy lights are a fabulous way to add a little extra theatre to the show. If you can, really go for it! Disco balls, lava lamps, candles …

Mirrors

Good use of mirrors is another great way to spice things up.

If you have any full-length mirrors, set them up in the room. As you dance, your partner will catch your reflection. Low and behold, he has two – or maybe even three – gorgeous creatures dancing for him all at once.

Tunes

Your choice of music is vital. It can make or break the atmosphere. Choose music that you both love. Make a compilation that will last the whole evening – not just while you're dancing. Talk about this together, and set it all up before the show begins. It will be worth it, I promise.

When choosing the music

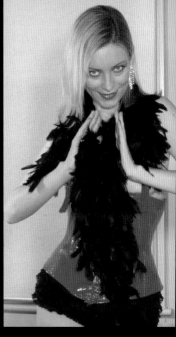

to dance to, go for something you know well. If there is one song that you love more than any other, give it a try to see if it is suitable. How does it make you feel? Does it inspire you? It's entirely up to you how many songs you perform to, although more than two can be quite exhausting.

If you want to create a classic striptease, choose music from the 40s and 50s. Old-fashioned jazz is really atmospheric. There are compilation CDs available now that are designed especially for performing this style of dance to.

For inspiration, listen to song lyrics. Maybe there is a song you love that has a special, meaningful lyric that would help you to choreograph your routine. Personally, I love to strip to slightly comical music. This is a fun dance, so let's have fun!

Final touches

When the evening of the date arrives, make sure your lover knows where you would like him to sit. If you've been rehearsing in front of a mirror, he should sit near to where your mirror has been, if possible. Otherwise, you'll have to alter your dance position, which can be disconcerting.

Finally, just before you change into your fabulous alter ego, do a quick check to make sure you have everything you're likely to need for the evening. You don't want to be nipping out to the shops all night – especially in that outfit!

Do you want to go for it? Do you really want your man to love your dance? Of course you do! To whet his appetite, in the days before the show

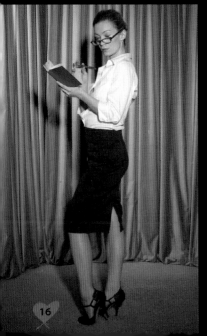

feed him little clues about what to expect. If you'll be dancing under the guise of a fantasy persona, tell your lover the name of the minx he'll meet. Mmm, the anticipation will be intoxicating.

Who will you be? His mistress, secretary, private dancer, a movie star …? Let your imagination go wild.

There is an element of acting involved in a great striptease. Try to become your chosen character. Allow her to infiltrate your mind. When I invent a character for my performances, I like to give her a history. She may be a

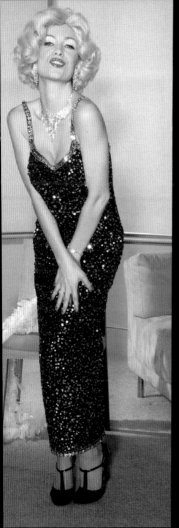

wild nymph who had a mysterious childhood spent living with gypsies; or perhaps she's a goddess from another universe; or maybe she's my lover's mistress, different to me in so many ways … I have a trigger in my mind that switches to a particular persona as soon as I start to dance.

You could build your costume around this great new you. How does she dress? Could you employ a theme that will add to the theatre of the show? What music will she like? Lose yourself in this fantasy world.

The most frequently asked question in my classes is, 'What should I wear?' To which I reply, 'You can do a fabulous strip from almost anything. Why, I bet you'd look stunning simply taking off your hat!'

The true you

Striptease can be so much fun. Relax and ask yourself, honestly, what you'll find enjoyable. You don't have to strip to your underwear or step outside your comfort zone in any way. Strictly speaking, striptease isn't about nudity. Professional dancers wear beautiful nipple tassels or pasties (nipple covers with no tassel) and spectacular frilly knickers, and these are kept on throughout the dance. They often wear corsets called 'waspies', too, to emphasize the waist.

Oh, the glamour

Of course, you should wear whatever makes you feel ultra-glamorous. Have a look to see what you have hiding away in your wardrobe. Maybe you'll rediscover a wig that you haven't worn for ages. What about those gorgeous stilettos you bought two years ago that are still in their box?

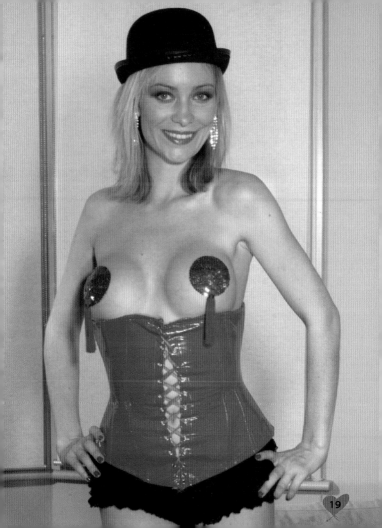

Have a look on the internet. Type 'Burlesque' and 'Striptease' into a search engine and see what you find. You should be able to get some simple but effective ideas.

A long dress always looks elegant, especially teamed with long black gloves. A feather boa is standard fair in a classic striptease, and it'll feel great against your skin – and his.

The only rule when it comes to clothing is that whatever you wear must be easy to take off. Avoid zips that you can't reach and hook-and-eye fastenings, except in bras.

High-heels are an essential part of any striptease routine.

I suspect that, from your lover's point of view, stockings and suspenders are vital, too.

Finishing touches

Give some thought to the little extras that can turn a good look into a stunning creation. Make-up is crucial – wear lots of it! It will give you so much extra confidence. Painted nails and beautiful jewellery will also add to your allure, and false eyelashes are devastatingly sexy.

Getting ready for your show is like preparing for a magical ritual. As you dress, imagine how beautiful you'll look as you glide elegantly across the room.

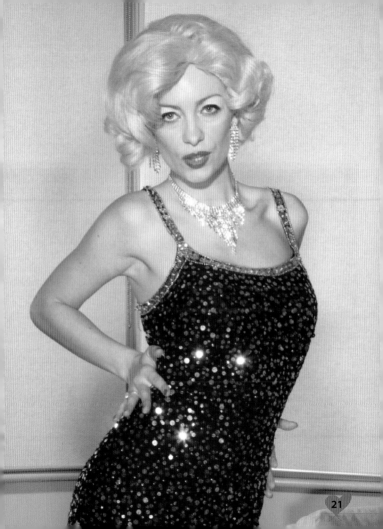

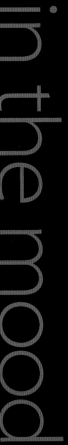

in the mood

Before we start learning the dance moves, let's sprinkle a little fairy dust around. This dance style relies more on atmosphere and mood than on dance routines. In this section I shall show you what I mean.

Facial expressions are a key factor. Whatever you're doing, think about the message being portrayed right there on your pretty face. Time to get your acting skills into shape!

There is a good deal of skill involved in taking off our clothes and dancing erotically at the same time. To help you perfect this art, I've included a striptease masterclass for you to follow. Good luck.

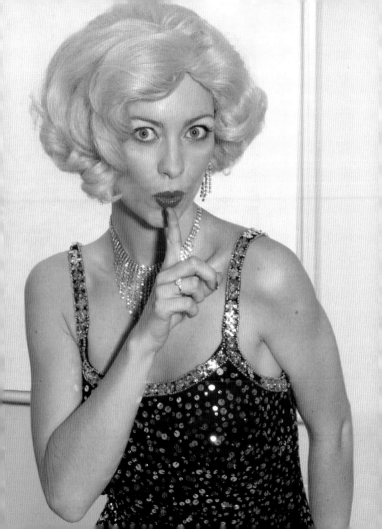

In striptease, the ultimate aim is to make our audience smile.

When you're smiling

If your face is dull, your dance will be dull. If your face looks bright and animated, your show will be spectacular.

When I was a professional striptease artist, I would say that about 90 per cent of my audience concentrated solely on my face. You can get away with anything if your face is sassy and engaging.

The most important expression is the sultry smile. Smiling while you dance sounds easy, but it's actually quite difficult. Unless you have a lot of dancing experience, remembering to smile along with everything else that you're trying to get right takes a lot of practice.

Try out your routine in front of a mirror as often as you can. Watch your face carefully and experiment with different expressions. See what a difference that smouldering smile makes!

Cheeky girl

Another classic striptease face is a little bit naughty and a little bit cheeky. Place your hand over your mouth and

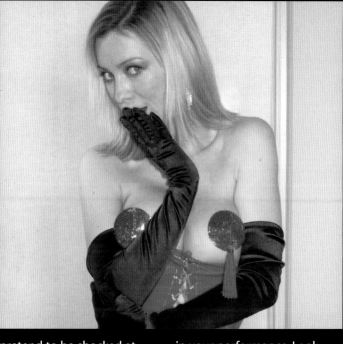

pretend to be shocked at your own naughtiness – this is great fun!

The eyes have it

It is worth remembering that your eyes can lead the drama in your performance. Look at your lover as much as you can. Hold him in your sexy gaze. Occasionally, look down at your body as though it's a glorious wonder. I promise that his eyes will follow.

There aren't many rules in striptease, which is why it can be so much fun. You may choose to dance in a stately, elegant way, or you could use quicker, more energetic movements. It all depends on the music you use.

Moves to lose

The only rule you really should remember is to be entertaining. Don't be drab and unconfident or lewd and undignified. And please don't get drunk before you dance; you will look awful and the whole experience will be embarrassing for you both.

Some ladies forget themselves, become a little overzealous and strip off far too quickly. The emphasis is on the tease, not the strip. Undress slowly.

Something else you should avoid is mouthing the words to the songs as you dance. Some people do, and it looks very strange!

Moves to use

Concentrate on moving beautifully. Even if you're just walking around, make sure you glide across the floor. Use the whole room as your stage. Turn your back on your lover

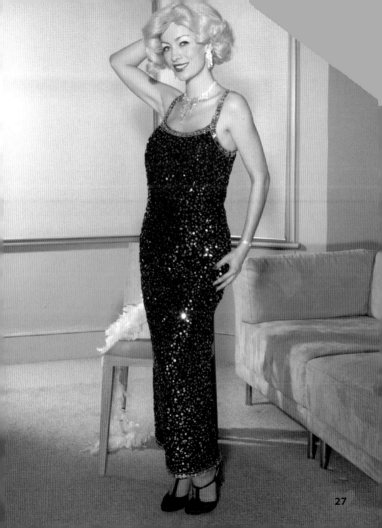

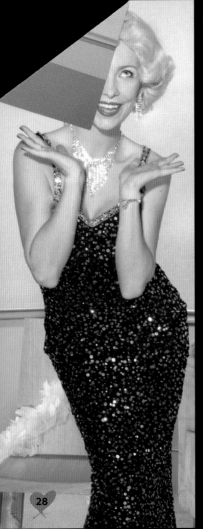

and walk away from him, then cheekily look back and shimmy that gorgeous bottom.

Open up your body language by moving your arms and hands gracefully. This will give you added confidence. Focus on your posture, keeping your head up and your shoulders back.

Follow the greats

For inspiration, watch some old striptease films, such as *Gypsy*, or some routines by the Hollywood movie director and musical choreographer, Busby Berkeley. Striptease is currently enjoying a renaissance, so there may be some shows in your area that you could go to see.

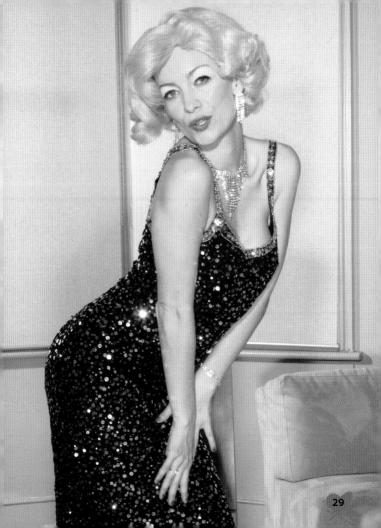

Well, ladies, the time has finally arrived. Put on some fabulous underwear and a gorgeous dress and stand in front of your mirror. We are going to S.T.R.I.P. – Sense; Tease; Reveal; Ignite; Parade!

Think sensual

Get your chosen music playing and start to dance sensuously. For now, we are just 'sensing' the timing of the song, so no elaborate dance steps just yet. I want you to get used to moving a little as you undress. Keep your head up and remember that smile!

Unzip When your music is about a third of the way through, begin to take off your dress. If you have a zip, undo it very slowly. Some dancers turn unzipping into an art form. Play with the zip,

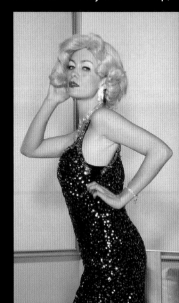

...awing it up and down a few times before unzipping it fully.

Disrobe If you have straps, remove them one by one using the opposite hand to shoulder. Let the dress slide to the floor. Step out of it sexily, pick it up, then throw it softly to one side.

Feel the suspense Don't take off your bra immediately. In the show you will want to 'tease' your lover a little. Allow yourself some time to show off your gorgeous underwear. He shouldn't know at this stage whether you're going to reveal more.

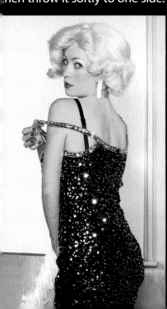

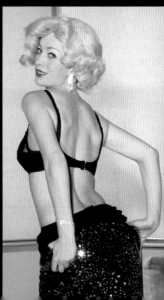

a play Sense how much music you have left. I suggest that you start to take off your bra about halfway through the song. This is why it's so important to know your music well. Now, turn your back to the mirror (this will be your over on the night) and undo the clasp. Holding the bra tight against your breasts with your arms, turn around to face the mirror. Begin to remove the straps from your shoulders. Take your time over this. It should look as though you are peeling off a layer of skin.

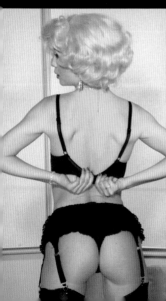

Aim to tease Continue to hold your bra in place – we don't want to reveal our beautiful tasselled nipples too soon! When you sense the time is right, turn away again, slip off your bra and throw it provocatively to one side – but keep your breasts covered with your hands or arms.

Reveal all Turn around again, look in your mirror and slowly, beautifully, slide away your hands to display your dazzling, bejewelled orbs. Are you smiling? This is the moment your lover will be waiting for!

Be a showgirl Now all the hard work is done, you can parade your fabulous self, and practise teasing your man with your cheeky show. Allow about a minute of the music for this part.

Wow – you've done it! Practise again and again, and, when you're ready, make that date!

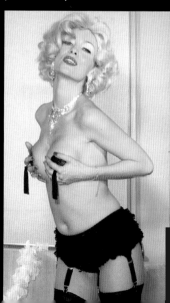

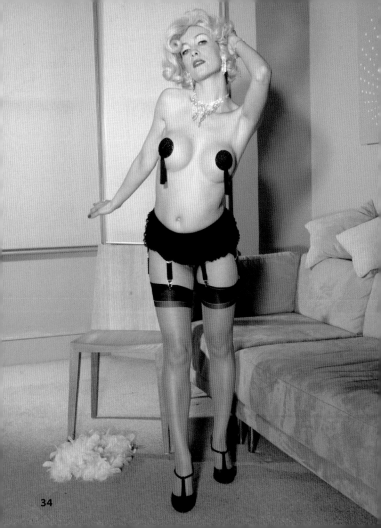

using props

To add a theatrical touch to your show, why not incorporate some props?

Striptease artists use all kinds of gimmicks and themes in their shows, some of them truly elaborate and brilliant. The scariest show I've seen involved a python. I'm afraid I can't give you any tips about that as I've never tried it!

In this book we will concentrate solely on the classics: long gloves, bowler hat, cane and feather boa. Please don't use them all in one show. Choose one or two and use them creatively. And don't forget to practise in front of that mirror.

Gloves can add a wonderfully erotic touch to a performance. There is a whole art form surrounding their removal. The classic striptease style is to begin your show by removing a glove. This looks great, but there is another reason behind it. It's much harder to take off a dress and a bra with gloves on!

Remove the glove on your dominant hand first (So, if you're left-handed, take off the left glove.) Begin by pulling each finger of the glove with your teeth or other hand to loosen it. Then gently glide it off. Let the glove fall into your lover's lap.

You can leave the other glove in place throughout the show if you wish, or take it off in the same way.

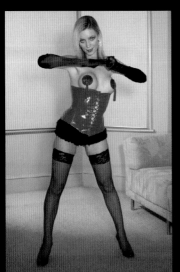

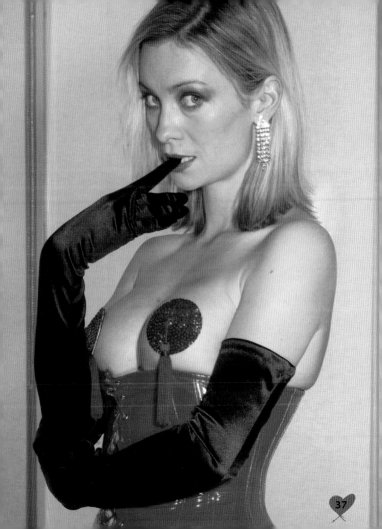

A bowler or top hat can look absolutely fantastic in a striptease. There are numerous ways to use it. You could simply leave it on throughout your striptease. It sounds too easy, I know, but being sexy isn't about tying yourself in knots. Just enjoy your props, and this means keeping within your comfort zones.

A classic trick is to take the hat off first – slowly, remember. Place it on the arm of a chair until you've just removed your bra and are still hiding your

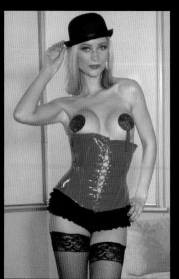
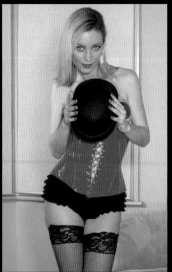

breasts with your hands. Turn your back to your lover, then place the hat over your breasts. Try tipping it forwards to reveal those gorgeous lovelies, then covering them again. As you turn your back to your audience, swap your hat from one hand to the other.

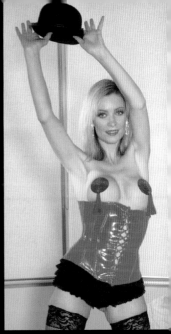

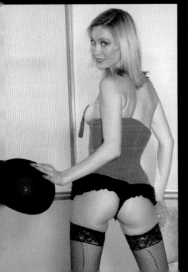

At the end of your show, slowly lift the hat above your head with both hands.

And for a final flourish, you could throw the hat to your man as you leave the stage!

cane

This is a sophisticated way to bring a little naughtiness into your show. If you use a cane well, nothing looks more elegant. But, the cane can be seen as a phallic object in striptease so we must be careful how we use it. You can be suggestive, but never lewd.

As you make your entrance, carry a cane under your arm. Then, when you turn to face your man, stand the cane on the floor in front of you, resting both your hands on top. A lovely slow wiggle of the bottom will look great at this point.

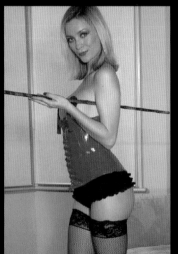
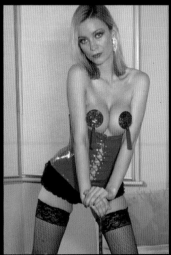

A nice little trick to try is to swing the top of the cane from one hand to the other, in time to the music.

Or, when your back is turned to your partner, hold the cane lengthways and bend forwards, brushing it across your bottom. Look back at your lover and give him a cheeky wink.

You may also use the cane to gently touch your man. Be careful, though. If you hurt him, he won't be impressed.

There are so many little movements you can do with a cane. Use your imagination, and your mirror, and see for yourself what works. For more inspiration watch the Fred Astaire movie, *Top Hat*.

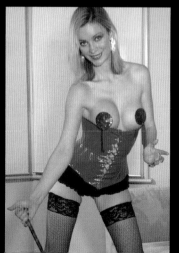
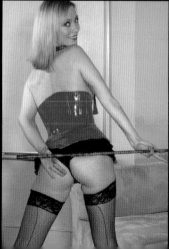

The good old boa is my particular favourite. I love the feeling of those feathers wrapped around my nearly naked flesh. Ooh, I quiver at the thought!

First, though, a warning: it is possible to get it very wrong with a boa, so be careful. If you're wearing a lot of finery, don't use it at the very beginning of your dance – you run the risk of looking a bit like an eccentric old lady. When you're preparing the stage before your show, drape your boa on a chair or table where you can pick it up easily later.

Just after you remove your bra, before you reveal your breasts, drape the boa around your shoulders and over your tasselled bosoms.

As you dance, allow the boa to reveal a breast occasionally, then cover it up again. Slowly, slowly, pull it away from your body and drape it around your lover's shoulders. Pull it sensuously at one end so that it glides across the back of his neck, over his body and onto the floor.

Turn and walk away, trailing the boa behind you as you leave … Oh, you tease!

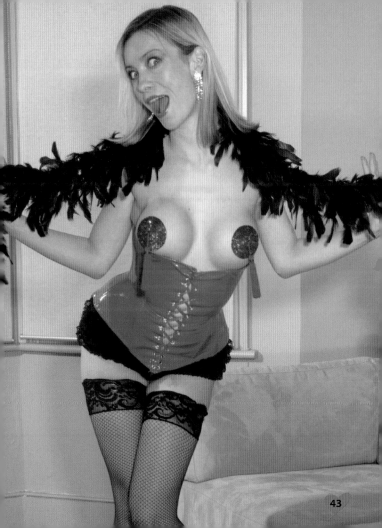

43

basic moves

I love to strip! Yes, ladies, I really do, and if you want to put on a great performance, this should be your mantra, too. Fall in love with your show. Enjoy the freedom of dancing for your partner on this magical evening.

Now that you're familiar with the concept, it's time to learn some of the basic steps used in striptease. There are lots of moves you can try; they're all really simple but very elegant.

Once you've mastered these steps, I hope you will feel inspired to experiment with some moves of your own. Remember, there are very few rules. As long as you undress

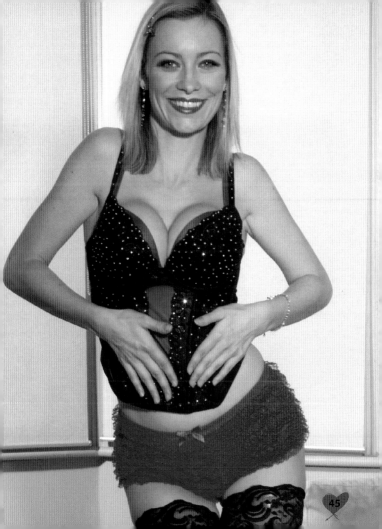

slowly and elegantly, remain gorgeous at all times and dance beautifully, you can do anything you want!

Striptease is about having fun with your audience. It should make them laugh. It isn't meant to be degrading or uncomfortable for anyone. A good strip show should leave your lover breathless and shouting for more.

I can't emphasize enough that this is your special night as well as your lover's. However you dance, it will be fabulous. Even if the worst happens – let's say you trip or get your costume stuck in your shoes – don't panic. Just stay calm, sort out the problem smoothly and with a twinkle in your eye, and carry on. Enjoy yourself.

If you forget your routine halfway through, improvise. I've seen artistes simply walk their way through a song. But because they were super-confident and had vibrant smiles on their faces, the audience didn't notice.

Be a confident goddess, a brave warrior and a loving partner and all will be well – I promise.

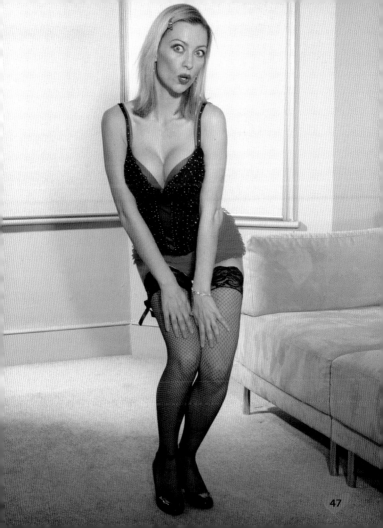

the walk

How you walk says a lot about your personality. Do you hold your head up or let it hang down? Do you race to your destination or shuffle along,

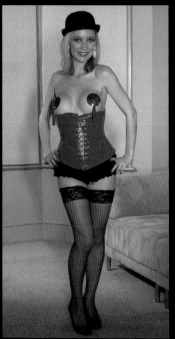

gazing at your surroundings? Your walk is your signature.

Your walk is the first thing we must get right. Imagine there is a golden chain attached to the top of your head and a magical force is controlling the other end, forcing you to walk with your head held up.

As you walk, relax your shoulders and straighten your back. Let your arms relax by your sides or run your fingers through your hair. Parade around to the music. How grand do you feel?

the figure eight

This movement has its roots in belly dancing. The sensuous sway of the hips is wonderfully erotic and will make your lover drool. It's most effective when performed slowly and with total eye contact. You'll make him melt with this one.

Begin with your feet together. Then move your hips so that your right hip draws a circle to the right, then the left hip draws a circle to the left. Accentuate your womanly curves by making the figure eight as large as possible.

As this is an Eastern dance move, try to incorporate a little Eastern promise with your arms. Visualize the way Indian dancers use their hands as they perform.

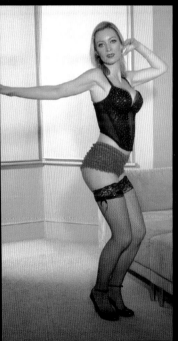

the shimmy

This beautiful movement is used in many exotic dance forms. It only really works when you're facing your partner, so, stand in front of that mirror again – let's witness the delights that await him.

Stand with your feet together, head up, shoulders back and relaxed. Slowly bend your knees and move your hips from side to side. Go down as far as you can. Keep your back straight as you bend. Then, slowly straighten your legs and return to standing. Either hold your arms out to the sides or touch your body and legs as you move.

This looks even more fabulous if you can shake your breasts at the same time. Go on, give it a try!

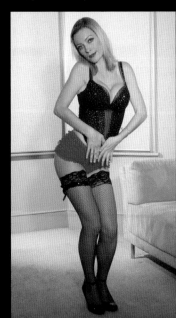

50

As we know, it's really quite difficult to remove your clothes while dancing. Performing complicated dance steps and fiddling around with a bra is almost impossible. This move is easy to perform, so it's perfect to use while you're taking off an item of clothing. You are free to focus on that troublesome clasp or zip.

Begin with your feet together or a few inches apart. Now, draw the biggest circle you can manage with your hips. Push your pelvis forwards as your hips come round to the front, and push your bottom back as your hips move to the back.

Perform this movement slowly. Allow its hypnotic power to drive your lover to distraction!

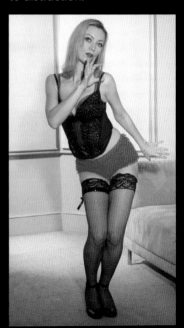

the turns

In striptease, we must believe that we're glorious beings. We demand to be admired and worshipped from every angle.

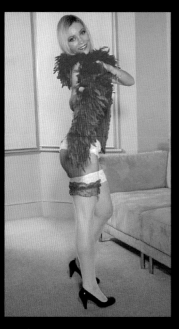

So, you must turn slowly so that your lover can see that you're totally scrumptious.

There are a number of ways to turn around as you dance. The easiest technique is to move your weight from one foot to the other as you gracefully turn on the spot. For an extra saucy touch, wiggle your posterior as you turn. Fabulous!

For a more adventurous variation, try turning as you walk. Simply step onto your right foot and pivot onto your left as you move. You may like to hold your hands sexily above your head as you turn.

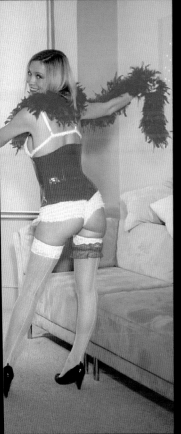

Keep your eyes on your lover throughout; flick your head around to meet his gaze.

You don't have to turn fully every time. Sometimes simply turn until you have your back to your man. As you look over your shoulder, tease him with a cheeky grin and a wink – and shake your booty! Give your bottom a gentle smack, too.

Vary the speed at which you turn. Try some slow, sensual moves and some quicker, more lively steps. Remain in charge of your body as you move and don't get carried away. Be elegant, magical and, above all, smile!

the dip

Almost like a bow, the dip has developed over time to encourage the audience to appreciate what we are doing. This slightly comical move can be performed facing your lover, to the side, or away from him. It works particularly well with the 'Ooh, aren't I naughty' expression illustrated on page 25.

Placing your hands on your knees, bend forwards from the hips. You can either stand with your feet together, a few inches apart or wide apart.

To add a comic edge, stand with your feet apart and face your man. Bend forwards, then, as you straighten up, turn your toes inwards and bend your knees towards each other. Cover your mouth with your hand and give him a cheeky wink!

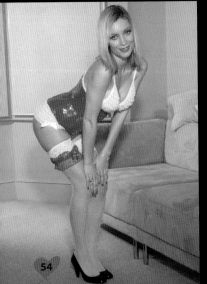

54

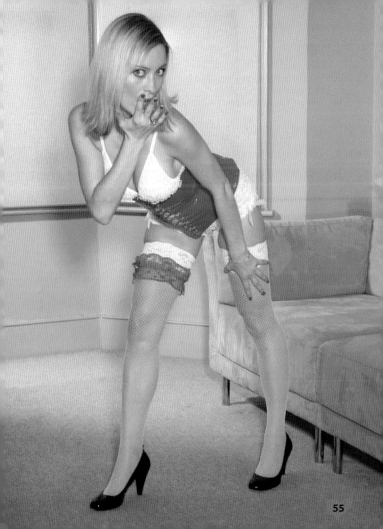

the shake

The shake is a real classic, and can be used very effectively throughout your show. There are two types of shake: one involving the bottom, and the other the bosom. I love them both as they're easy to do and always make people smile.

We'll start with the bottom shake. Stand with your back to your lover and shake your gorgeous derrière as fast as you can, keeping the shoulders still. Try to isolate your bum.

Now, facing your audience, isolate your breasts in the same way and give them a really good shake. It helps to hold your arms out to the sides. If you're topless and are blessed in the bosom department, do be careful – this can hurt. Practise in the mirror until you look utterly fabulous.

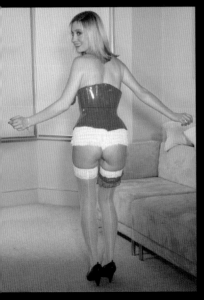

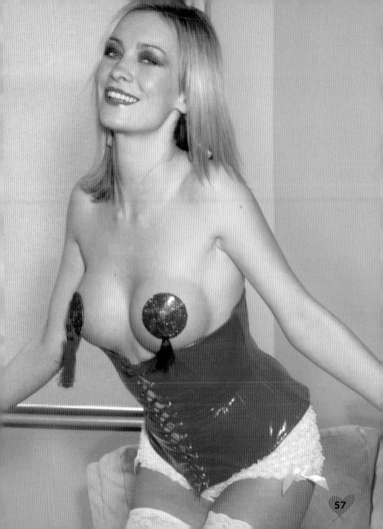

chair moves

One of the most popular props, and the most readily available, is the dining chair.

Before the show, position your chair at least 1.5 metres (5 feet) from where your partner will sit. You need room to dance all the way around it. Make sure the chair you use is solid and well made. We don't want any accidents.

When it comes to the chair moves, you can be as brazen or as prim as you like. You may want to simulate sexual moves, move the chair as you dance or simply sit on it elegantly.

For further inspiration, try watching Liza Minnelli in the film *Cabaret*, or Catherine Zeta Jones in *Chicago*.

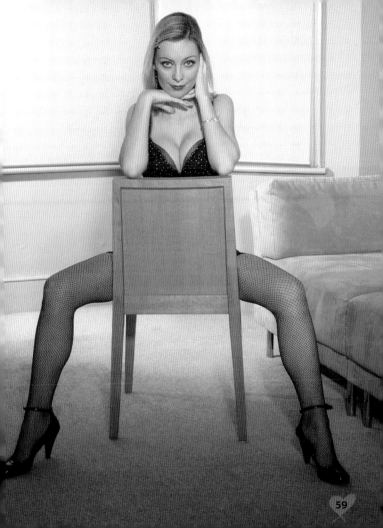

As you dance, try to be aware of where the chair is placed. It looks a little awkward if you have to look behind you before you sit down. When you're ready to sit, step in front of the chair, bend your knees and slowly lower yourself onto the seat. Keep your back really straight and don't lean back in the chair. And keep your knees together, like a good girl. From this position there are a number of moves you can try. Here are some suggestions.

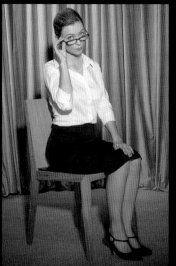

Knee tease

Place your hands on your knees and push your legs wide apart. Wait a moment, then close them again. This is a great move to use early in the show when you're still wearing most of your clothes,

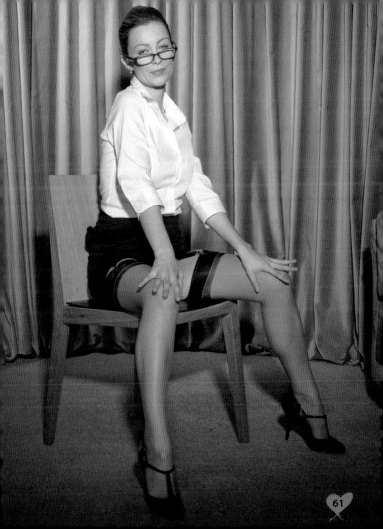

as it allows your audience a quick glimpse of what he'll see more of later. Saucy!

Drive him wild
Push your bottom to the edge of the chair and lean back. Straighten one or both legs out in front of you and let your head fall back as though you're in total ecstasy. If your hair is loose, run your fingers through it sexily. Yeah!

Chair straddle
Straddling the chair always looks gorgeous. Once you're in position, gently lift your bottom up and down or circle your hips, simulating lovely things. Oh my! You can do this facing towards or away from your lover – depending on how cheeky you're feeling!

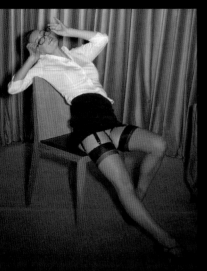

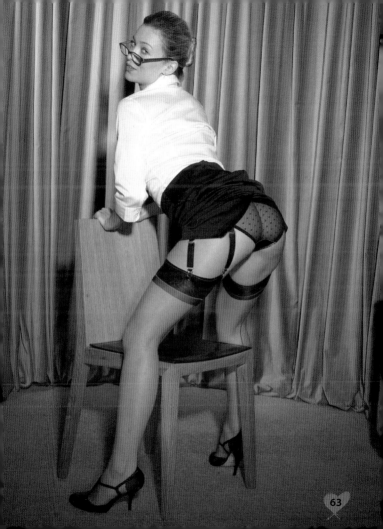

Well, it wouldn't be a chair dance without a few kicks thrown in here and there, would it?

Single-leg kick

Sitting comfortably facing your man, grip the sides of the seat for support. Lift your right

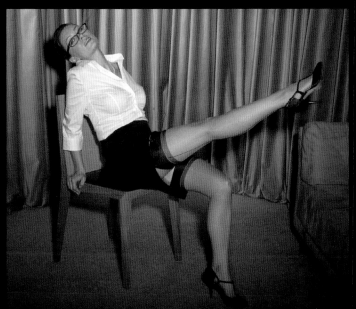

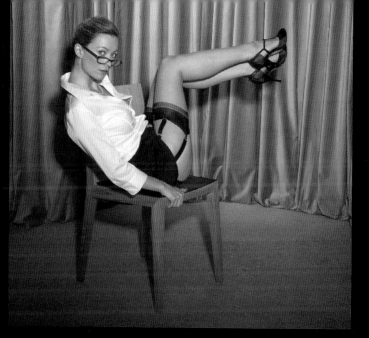

leg and kick to the left. Then lift your left leg and kick to the right.

Twist and kick

This is another great kick. Grasp the seat as before. Then lift both legs out in front of you and twist them to the left. Lift both legs as high as you can. Then repeat to the right. To make this move a little easier, lean back in the chair as you kick.

Bending and stretching yourself over, or on, a chair can look fabulous. You don't have to limit these moves to the dining chair. You could use the sofa or any other chair that is close to your dance space. These are a few of the bends I have used, but, remember to use your imagination and let the ideas flow.

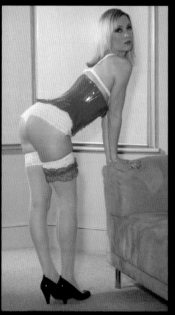

Bend and shake

Stand in front of your chair with your back to the audience. Place your feet together or wide apart. Keeping your knees straight, lower your upper body and hold on to the sides of the chair seat or the arm of the sofa. Now, look back, wink and wiggle your booty. Gorgeous!

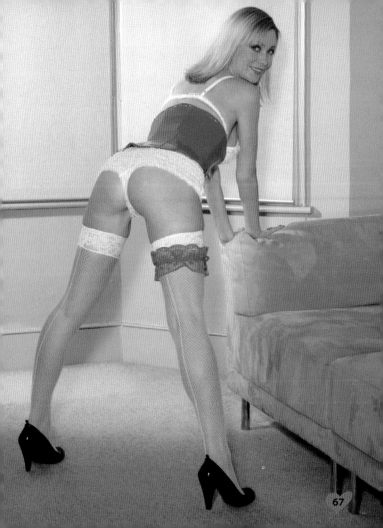

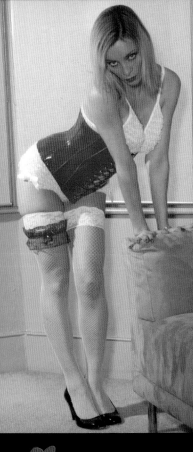

Bend and squeeze

Stand behind your chair, facing your lover. Place your hands on the chair back or the arm of the sofa. Put your feet together and lower your upper body forwards. Squeeze your cleavage together with your upper arms as you look longingly at your man. Mmm.

Bend and stroke

Stand to the left of your chair and face your audience. Place your right foot on the chair seat. Then bend forwards and slowly stroke all the way along your shoe, up your leg and along that beautiful thigh until your upper body is upright again. Lovely.

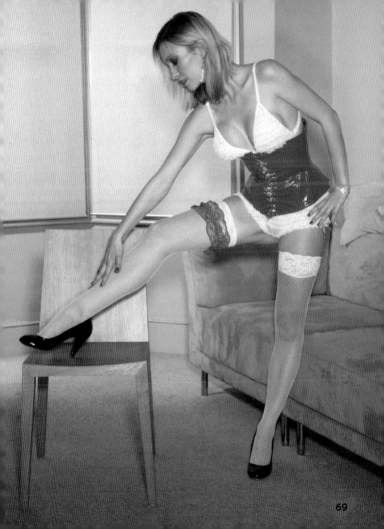

poses

Pausing is a very important element of dance. It can be quite boring to watch someone race through a routine. By striking a great pose and holding it for a few seconds you will add an extra element of excitement to your show. It will also provide a welcome opportunity to catch your breath.

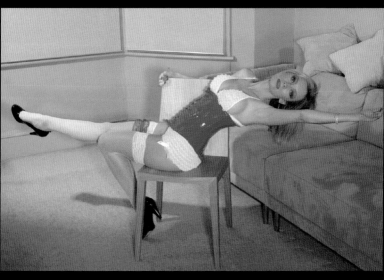

This is just one of the many stunning poses you could try. You'll need a dining chair with no arms. Stand with your back to the side of the chair and sit down so that you're sideways-on to your partner. Holding on to the back of the chair with one arm, lean back, bringing the other arm over your head in an arc. To extend this pose, lean back as far as you can and lift one leg out in front of you.

If you want to be really daring, stand on the chair, facing your partner. Lean forwards slightly and blow him a soft, slow kiss.

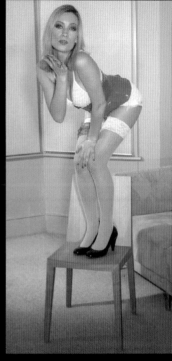

Any of the chair moves that I've shown you can make a great pose. Simply stop and hold your position every now and again.

the striptease

Ladies, you've stripped in front of a mirror, and you've learnt the moves. Now it's time to put your new skills together.

This simple routine is easy to follow; however, I would suggest that, to begin with, you practise it in stages. Take the first few steps and rehearse them repeatedly until you can link them together with ease. Then move onto the next part and do the same again.

As you know, props are a vital part of a great show. Here, I use a chair and a feather boa, but please use the props you most enjoy working with. There are lots to choose from, so try out a

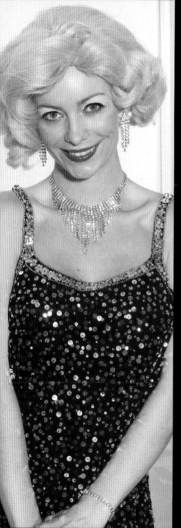

different combination each time you perform. Whatever you choose, if you won't be using it from the start, place it on your stage before the show.

As with any dance, timing is crucial. You're not only learning how to perform the routine, but also how to sense the timing in your music. Choosing a song that you adore will give you extra motivation to put on a spectacular show. So, cue the music and get rehearsing.

Once you've learnt this routine, I hope you will feel confident enough to put together your own show. There's no stopping you now, baby!

For immediate impact, try to make a spectacular entrance into the room. As soon as your music begins, walk, like a Vegas showgirl, into the centre of your stage. Remember that gold chain that is helping you to walk so powerfully (*see page 48*). You don't have to move quickly. Just glide across the floor beautifully. Stop just in front of the chair.

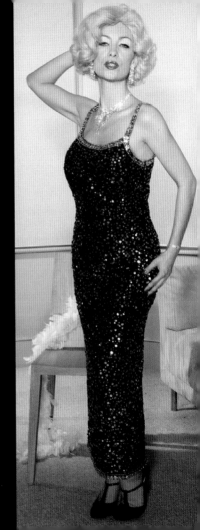

Turn to face your audience and circle your hips. Smile and run your fingers through your hair in a coquettish, come-hither manner.

Begin to turn slowly, keeping your eyes on your lover for as long as you can. Turn all the way round to display every aspect of your outfit to your audience.

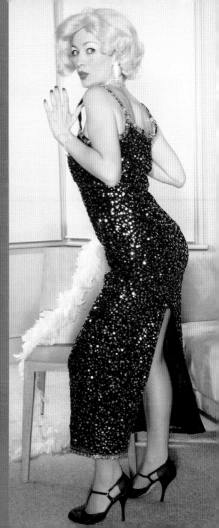

Sit down on the chair, keeping your legs and feet together. Keep your back very straight and place your hands on your knees. Pretending to be really prim, put one hand over your mouth in mock surprise at your own cheekiness.

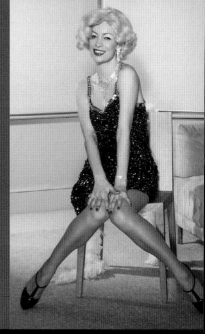

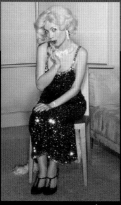

If your dress is long, slowly pull it up to show off your knees. Place both hands on your knees and push them open until they are wide apart. Allow a second or two to pass, then push your legs back together.

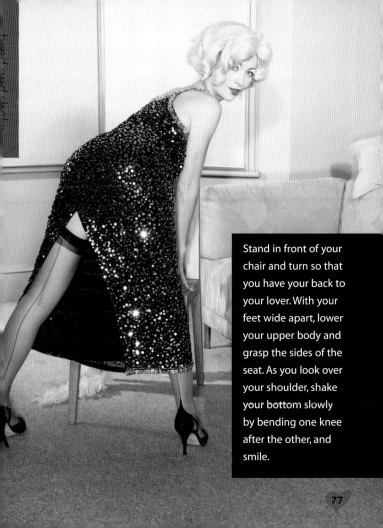

Stand in front of your chair and turn so that you have your back to your lover. With your feet wide apart, lower your upper body and grasp the sides of the seat. As you look over your shoulder, shake your bottom slowly by bending one knee after the other, and smile.

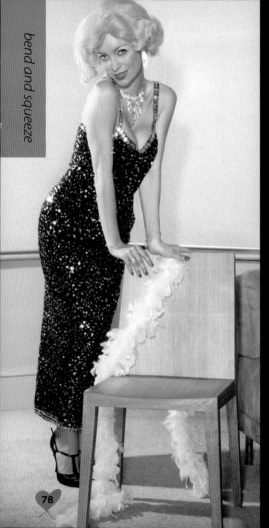

Stand up straight, walk
around to the back of
the chair and turn to
face your man. Resting
your hands on the
chair back, lean
forwards and, with
your upper arms,
press your cleavage
together. Hold this
pose for a few seconds.
 Walk gracefully to
the side of your chair
so that you have some
free space. Turn fully
as you walk.

As you turn to face your audience once more, place your feet together and create a figure eight with your hips. Hold your hands up in sweet abandon as you hypnotize your lover with your sumptuous hips.

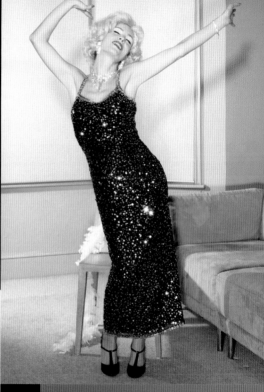

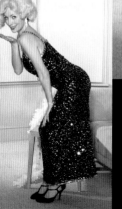

the dip

Turn a little so that you're in profile to your audience, and dip down with your hands on your knees. Give your man a lovely big smile, and blow him a kiss.

79

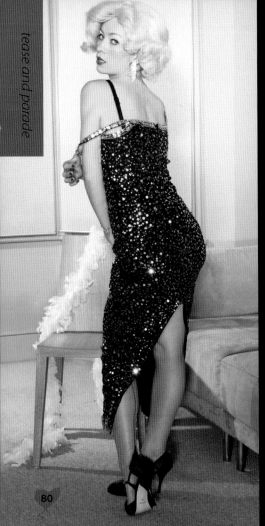

Now, let's begin to tease. Stand straight, circle your hips slowly and peel off one shoulder strap. You may play naughtily with your zip, but don't go any further just yet!

Parade and strut your funky stuff around the room, changing the direction of your walk with gorgeous, elegant turns. Caress your figure as you move and keep your eyes on your man as much as possible. You are the predator in this dance – behave like one!

When your music is about a third of the way through, it's time to remove your dress. Standing still, peel off the other shoulder strap. Slowly tease down the zip and allow your dress to fall to the floor.

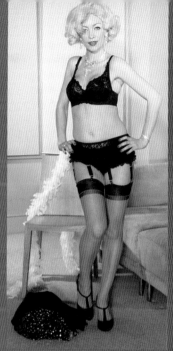

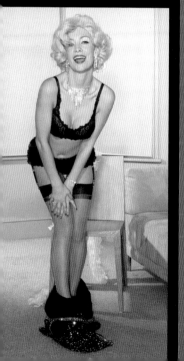

Slowly step out of the dress. Bend down sexily to pick it up, then drop it on the chair beside your partner. See what happens …

Now you are in your gorgeous underwear. Allow your lover to see you, to really drink in this beautiful sight. Stand in front of your chair, facing him, and shimmy down, bending your knees. Shimmy that lovely bosom as you go.

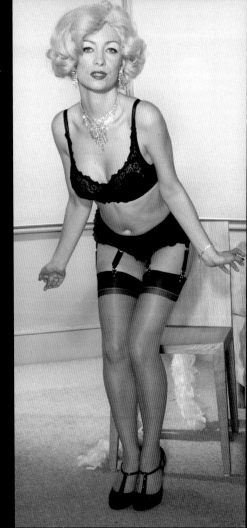

Sit down on the chair, facing your audience, and grasp the sides of the seat. Slowly raise your right leg and kick out to the left, then lift your left leg and kick to the right.

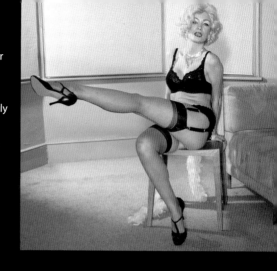

Slide yourself around on the chair so your lover can see you in profile. Hold on to the back of the chair with one arm, lean back and kick up both legs. Throw your right arm back in an arc.

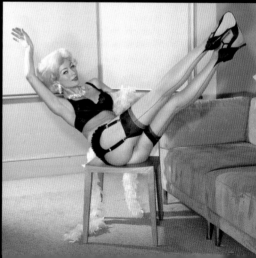

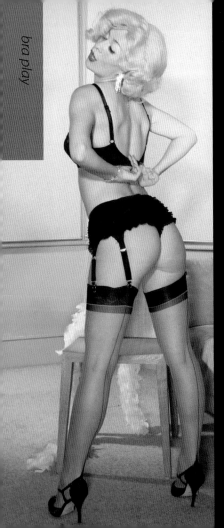

Lower your feet to the floor and stand up. Now, let's take off that bra! Turn away from your audience so that your lovely back is on show. If you can, look over your shoulder sensuously as you undo your bra hooks.

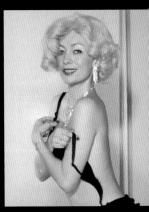

Holding your bra in place with your arms, turn to the side and remove just one bra strap.

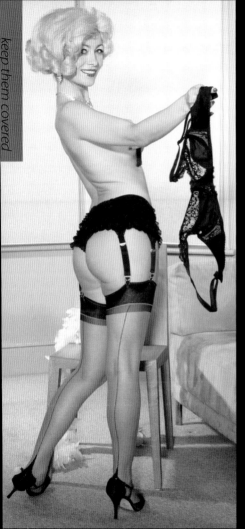

Parade around, strut your stuff, do anything you like, but keep hold of your bra with your hands.

Standing beside the chair, place your right foot on the seat. Bend your left leg up and down to make those amazing hips wiggle.

Walk away from your partner, looking back as you go. Now, it's time to discard your bra. Slip it off completely, keeping your breasts covered with your hands. Throw the bra away from your dance space.

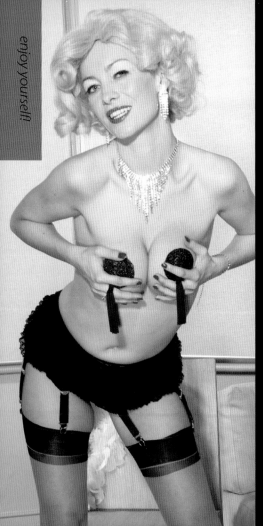

enjoy yourself!

Still standing with your back to your audience, perform another little shimmy. Really tease him. Don't take your hands away from your tasselled beauties yet.

Turn to face your man, dip by bending forwards from the hips, then turn and walk away from him.

Covering your breasts with one arm, slowly drag the boa from the chair. Turn away from your man to drape it seductively over your shoulders and breasts. Then turn and walk towards him.

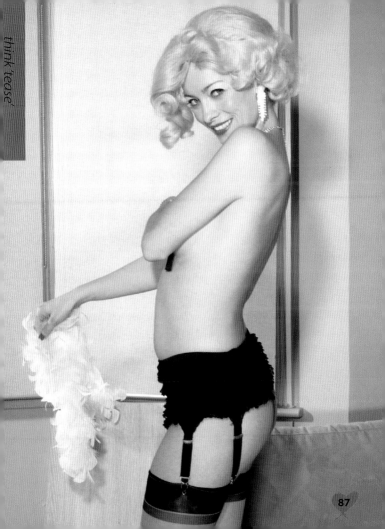

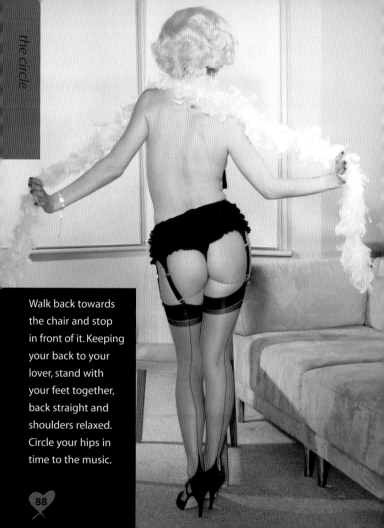

Walk back towards
the chair and stop
in front of it. Keeping
your back to your
lover, stand with
your feet together,
back straight and
shoulders relaxed.
Circle your hips in
time to the music.

88

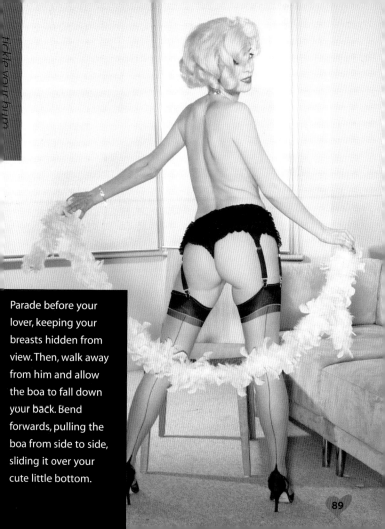

Parade before your lover, keeping your breasts hidden from view. Then, walk away from him and allow the boa to fall down your back. Bend forwards, pulling the boa from side to side, sliding it over your cute little bottom.

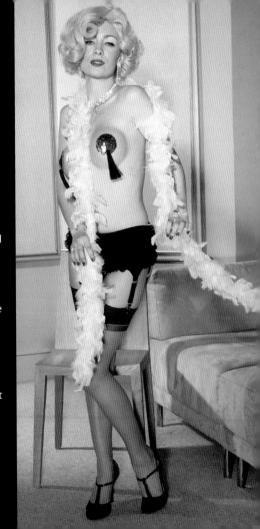

Place the boa round
your shoulders and
over your beautiful
bosom. Turn to face
your man. Now, give
him a cheeky little
glimpse of one
breast under the
boa. Quickly cover
it again, then repeat
with the other one.
This will drive your
lover wild!

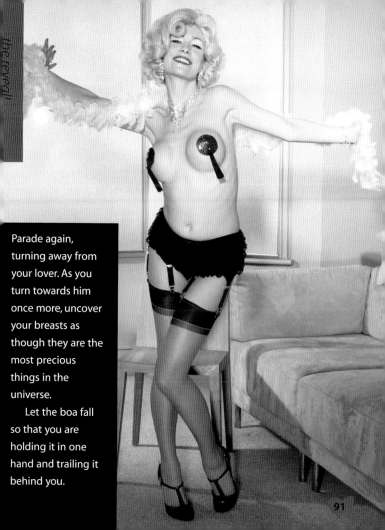

Parade again,
turning away from
your lover. As you
turn towards him
once more, uncover
your breasts as
though they are the
most precious
things in the
universe.

Let the boa fall
so that you are
holding it in one
hand and trailing it
behind you.

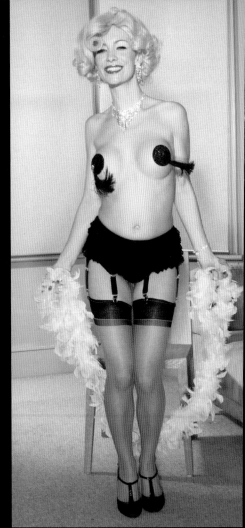

After this slow reveal, shall we make him smile? Come on, let's do the shake. Bend your knees slightly and shake 'em, baby, shake!

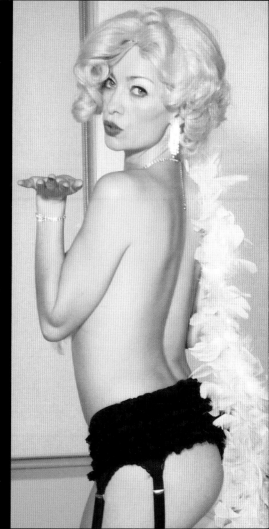

The hard work is done. You can walk around, flaunting your newfound confidence. Just before the end of the show, walk towards your man and drape the boa over his knees.

Then, to finish, walk away, gently pulling the boa away from him again. Blow him a little kiss, give him a wink and strut your funky ass out of there.

Leave him begging for more!

If I wear suspenders and stockings, should I take those off, too?
No. Absolutely not. Leave them on for your man to drool over. Striptease is about teasing, not nudity.

How long should my show last?
I suggest between four and eight minutes. One to two songs is usually enough. Stay within your own comfort zone.

What if my partner laughs at me?
Laugh with him. This is supposed to be fun for you both. Don't be afraid to be entertaining. If he really loves you, he will be laughing in an encouraging way. If you feel uncomfortable, just stop. It isn't the end of the world.

How old is too old?
Never! Get yourself a gorgeous outfit, have your hair done and start practising. The only thing that matters is that you and your partner enjoy yourselves.

Do I have to be slim to perform a striptease?
No way! Some of my favourite striptease performers are larger ladies. Everybody's eyes light up when a real woman appears on stage. There's all the more to adore and love. Shake that voluptuous booty, baby!

What if I make a mistake?
If you rehearse as much as you can, all will be well. Your partner won't know if you go wrong unless you stop or look sheepish. Keep smiling and walking and he'll never suspect that anything has gone awry.

Where can I find ideas for shows?
Look inside yourself. Who do you want to be for a night? A nymph, an empress, a bunny girl? Live out your fantasies. There's an abundance of ideas everywhere you look. Be creative. Try asking your lover for ideas. What an eye opener that could turn out to be …

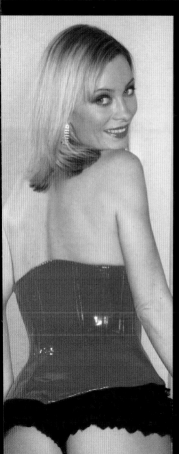

Well, ladies, I hope you feel a little more confident about striptease, now. Remember that you can do almost anything while stripping as long as it's elegant and self-assured. I've performed striptease routines all over the world as well as at home for my partner. I've made people laugh, I've turned them on, made them think – and once, I even made someone cry …

If you want to have a real giggle as you practise, and build confidence at the same time, why not ask a girlfriend to come over one night. You can perform your lovely routine for her, and, maybe even teach her a few moves. Whatever you do, do it because you want to, and have a blast!

*If you still feel insecure about your dancing, private or small group
lessons with Rebecca can be arranged through her website,
www.sevenveilsproductions.co.uk.*

About the Author

Rebecca Drury trained with the Royal Academy of Dance for twelve
years. During her time at university studying Performance Art, she
became a professional dancer and travelled internationally
performing lap dancing, pole dancing, striptease, the cancan,
the Dance of the Seven Veils and burlesque. In 2002, she was
nominated for Erotic Artist of the Year by the Leydig Trust.
She now runs a school teaching exotic dance, and is one of the
most successful teachers in the UK. Rebecca is the author of two
other *Naughty Girl's Guide* titles – *Lap Dancing* and *Pole Dancing*.
She lives in Brighton, UK, where she is renowned for her soirees
and nightclub events.

Acknowledgements

With thanks to Robert Smith for first seeing the potential of this
book, and Eddison Sadd for their help in making the book possible.
Thanks to Will for being my best friend. Thanks also to Moonie King,
Alistair Hughes and Sophia Acha for their patience. And thank you
to Annie Taylor at sirens_candybar@hotmail.co.uk for her beautiful
corsets, tassels and garters.